Dyslexia

A guide for teachers and parents

Dyslexia

A guide for teachers and parents

Margaret Newton
Michael Thomson

 University of London Press Ltd

'Reading maketh a full man,
Conference a ready man,
And writing an exact man'

Francis Bacon

'The world cheats those who cannot read'

IXth Century Chinese Poet

ISBN 0 340 20049 9

University of London Press Ltd.
St. Paul's House, Warwick Lane, London EC4P 4AH

Printed in Great Britain by
Elliott Brothers & Yeoman Ltd., Liverpool L24 9JL

Preface

This book is the result of many years experience in education and developmental psychology. It has been prepared in the Language Development Study Centre of the Applied Psychology Department of the University of Aston in Birmingham.

During the last eight years intensive effort has been directed at the Centre into the understanding and prediction of the primary (intrinsic) category of written language difficulty described by many specialists as Dyslexia. Children attend a weekly diagnostic and advisory clinic; teachers and other professionals attend the Centre for meetings and short conferences. Members of the Centre visit other establishments and parent-groups throughout the country to lecture and exchange findings on this type of learning failure. An indexing system of relevant publications has been started and is part of the continuing work of the Centre.

From all these activities has arisen the need for some kind of structured guide to the teaching of the dyslexic person. Just as an earlier guide to Dyslexia (Newton 1973) was written in response to requests from anxious parents and teachers, so it has been expanded and the present volume produced to meet a similar demand at the present time for actual techniques of teaching. Many of these techniques are already in use by able teachers throughout the country. They are brought together in this one small volume to serve as guidelines to many others who, having recognised the problem, are anxiously seeking advice on what to do next. We hope that the following pages will provide a basis for continuing investigation and understanding of this very real educational problem.

We should like to thank all members of the Language Development Study Team for their specific contributions and our Professor, Tom Singleton, who, by his tolerance of our ideas and beliefs, has made all this work possible. We gratefully acknowledge help given to us by The William Cadbury Trust and especially the personal interest of John Cadbury. Our thanks are also due to The Baring Foundation, J. A. Pye, The Lord Austin Trust, The Cole Charitable Trust and The Ratcliffe Foundation, whose financial support ensures continuity of the research programme.

Margaret Newton
Michael Thomson

Contents

PART 1
First Considerations

1. The nature of the problem

Collins (1967) wrote that remedial teaching is, in fact, first good teaching. Children with dyslexic-type written-language difficulties need a special kind of 'good teaching' if they are to acquire the skills they will need to take part in a verbally-based educational system. Moreover, the appropriate 'good teaching' must be set in a proper frame of reference. This would include consideration of the following three areas:

1. The specific developmental pattern of the individual dyslexic child.
2. The nature of the skill to be learned.
3. The way in which this skill can best be transmitted to match the unique learning patterns of the dyslexic child.

Before techniques are described, therefore, these three aspects of the problem will first be discussed.

2. Developmental learning patterns

Children vary greatly in maturational levels. Progress in intellectual, emotional, physical and social growth patterns is unique to each child, although based on general developmental sequences. There appears to be a readiness time for each child to learn, accept, understand and perform the various behaviours and skills demanded by society. Reading, spelling and writing are such skills. Normally, good teaching has its maximum effect when the complex variables involved in learning 'make sense'. Developing patterns of growth and experience from home and society influence this 'readiness' time.

Individual variations in intellectual growth patterns have been recognised since the turn of the century (Binet and Simon 1905). These differences in general underlying ability have been related to school-learning potential and teachers in general are aware of such factors; for example, the problems of the slow-learning child not yet ready for formal, symbolic material or of the very able child whose considerable ability is not recognised and developed.

In addition, the roles of home and society, i.e. the extrinsic, environmental factors, can present barriers to learning. Such barriers could be emotional in origin; for example, acute anxiety following upon some traumatic family event. A child can be blocked from learning by such events as sibling rivalry (e.g. the birth of a baby sister just as a five-year-old boy is about to begin school), by over-anxious and stressful parents, by feelings of rejection, by death in the family and by perceived difficulties in parental relationships. Secondary emotional stress is often experienced too as a result of school failure, when the child reaches the age of seven, eight or nine years without fulfilling the expectations of the peer group in written skills.

Socio-cultural barriers to learning are the subject of much present-day research. The so-called culturally deprived child is said to lack preparation in language skills, in life experiences, in person-oriented styles of rearing; whereas the culturally favoured child arrives at school well prepared with relevant experiences, to engage fully in the educational system.

The learning barriers could be in the school situation itself—over-large classes, especially at a time when a young child still needs a facilitating, supportive one-to-one relationship in which to begin new learning; inadequately prepared teachers, especially in the field of reading, spelling and fluent writing; changes of school and changes of teacher, preventing a continuity of meaningful learning; inappropriate teaching schemes.

The effects of all these environmental factors on learning to read are described by Schonell (1942) and Vernon (1957). Indeed Tizard (1972), chairman of the Advisory Committee on Handicapped Children, stresses these factors and prefers the term 'specific reading difficulties' to that of 'dyslexia' when referring to severe reading retardation. After at least forty years, however, since Gates and Bond (1936) and Nancy Catty (1933), this rather general term fails to give any helpful or diagnostic insight to practising teachers.

Remedial education during the past twenty-five years, especially in Great Britain, has been organised mainly within this framework of either extrinsic causation or intellectual retardation. Treatment has been based in a therapeutic context, individual and child-centred. The aim has been to relieve the anxiety of the child by rapport —therapy and play-therapy; to modify the home background if possible—in a clinical situation by the intervention of the psychiatric social worker; and to provide a well sequenced, well informed programme of remedial teaching. Such a model is exemplified by studies carried out in the Child Study Centre at the School of Education, Birmingham University. This centre was originally known as the Remedial Education Centre. It was set up in 1948 by Professor (later Sir) Fred Schonell in collaboration

3

with Dr (later Professor) Bill Wall. The Centre fulfilled the roles of research, treatment of children and the training of experienced teachers in the above techniques of treatment. Mia Kellmer-Pringle, the eminent educational psychologist, who was at one time responsible for direction of the Centre, wrote in 1952:

> The problem of educational retardation of children who are of average or very good ability is not only a serious educational, but also a social problem. Their underfunctioning means a loss of efficiency and a waste of ability now and in the future which the country can ill afford. More important still, the children themselves suffer and if offered no help become sooner or later serious emotional problems. The fact that the great majority of juvenile delinquents are educationally retarded shows how failure to derive emotional satisfaction at school may well be an important factor in directing children's energies into anti-social channels. By research into this problem, by training teachers to specialise in this work and by informal contacts with schools, the Centre aims at increasing awareness of this problem and at stimulating Educational Authorities to set up similar services in their areas.

3. The emergence of a primary factor

Such training programmes have exerted a strong influence on many present-day teachers and psychologists who diagnose and treat within these terms of reference. The powers of the environment and intellect have been recognised by these specialists. Yet to some present-day research workers these barriers would, in some cases, be seen as secondary factors. A prime factor, involving intrinsic developmental patterns, has been isolated and described by many neurologists and neuro-psychologists. This factor is neurological in origin and involves individual differences in the development of sensory mechanisms (i.e. visual and auditory perception), motor mechanisms (especially handedness) and laterality of the brain hemispheres for language function (Zangwill 1960, Newton 1968). When there is unevenness of development between these functions and/or symmetrical, ambilateral function in place of dominance, difficulties of unstable perceptual patterns can arise which prevent the consistent learning of order and direction—visually, auditorily and graphically, in any one mode or in any combination of modes (Orton 1937). Sometimes the consequent difficulty in 'symbolia' or 'flash of recognition' is a result of 'maturational lag'; it will be resolved, at eight, nine, or ten years or at some later stage. It is often a genetic, familial growth pattern, seen in other family members (Critchley 1970, Hallgren 1950). Sometimes it is a condition caused by an 'at-risk' birth situation, pre-, peri-, or post-natal in origin (Kawi and Pasamanick 1959). Or it can be an interaction of both causes. It has been estimated on a probability distribution amongst the population that as many as 28 per cent of children entering school could be at risk within this category, minimally to grossly involved (Newton 1974). Observable signs in the individual child who has inconsistent sensory, motor and language functions can be discrepant patterns of left/right, eye, hand, ear, foot organisation. Orton (1937) described these as manifestations of the lack of cerebral dominance—'the child looks at random; cannot acquire series'. In cases where the above environmental or intellectual stresses are *also* present, formidable barriers against ordered, symbolic learning must be overcome, especially at the very young developmental age of five years.

4. Defining the category
This category of learning difficulty is often described at

the present time as 'dyslexia' or 'dyslexic-type language difficulty', from the original Greek—difficulty with the lexicon, the word. Dyslexia has been defined by the World Federation of Neurology (Critchley 1970) as 'a language disorder in children who, despite conventional classroom experience, fail to attain language skills of reading, writing and spelling commensurate with their intellectual abilities'. Confusion has arisen between educationists and neurologists owing to the use by the latter of the term 'word-blind' as a synonym for dyslexia. To the educationist this term represents an irretrievable, irremediable situation and is unacceptable; thus the very existence of this type of individual development pattern seems often to be disregarded, owing to the terminology used to describe it. But ambilateral types of language, sensory and motor functions are a reality despite differences in labelling and are incompatible with the nature of the skill to be learned, i.e. a written language system. This will be discussed, therefore, in the following section.

5. The nature of the skill to be learned

Written English is based on an alphabet of twenty-six letters. These letters are represented by a set of 'line drawings' (Gibson 1965) arbitrarily determined to represent the 'phonemes' or sounds of speech. Speech sounds (phonemes) are represented by arbitrary symbols (graphemes). These, unlike picture writing or the Chinese pictogram (word writing), are symbolic and unrelated to the actual event in the environment. The alphabet system is then expanded into word patterns (sequences of phoneme contrasts) and also spelling patterns (sequences of grapheme contrasts). Written language is thus sequential, in that letters and words must be put into a sequence. The letters (and words) must also be put into a correct order, in the sense that 'cat', when the order is changed, becomes 'act', a different meaning, but with the same constituent letters. Written language is also directional, in that letters have mirror-images: e.g. b, d; p, q; m, w; and so on. Thus letters must be correct directionally; 'cnd' is not 'cup', whereas if the event itself (a cup) is turned around, upside down, etc., it remains the same. Thus, to succeed in written language, symbols must be related to an event, and *perceived*, *stored* and *reproduced* consistently in visual, auditory and motor activities. It can be seen therefore that the system is characterised by rules, regularities, order, direction and sequence. It must therefore be *learned*. In order to learn the rules and techniques and relate them to required meaning, every letter, syllable, word, phrase, sentence must be perceived in exact form: 'het god saw no teh ded', although containing the required number of letters and correct word lengths, does not convey the meaning 'the dog was on the bed', The 'line-drawings' are often the mirror-image of each other: b, d; p. q; w, m; n, u. Recent evidence (Zangwill 1973) suggests that if the word 'doll' is scanned by a left-eye dominant child, the message received by the brain could be 'llob', which bears no relation to the teacher's reinforcing sound pattern 'doll'. Many words have mirror-image forms: was, saw; on, no; or possible internal re-arrangement: bird, brid; girl, gril. There is a left/right direction across the page, both to read and to write, and an ordered line progression down the page. So to perceive these patterns consistently and transmit them to the brain, a matching consistency of sensory mechanism activity is essential. The brain can only organise the message transmitted to it by the receptors. If consistently ordered patterns, exact representations of reality, are not transmitted, no exact engrams (or memory traces) are stored and so cannot therefore be retained and retrieved in meaningful form. The consequent muddle to the young learner is characterised by reversals,

7

mirror-images, bizarre spelling, slow, regressive reading patterns, inability to acquire written fluency, to use punctuation, to acquire the rules of syntax, or even the total inability to learn to read. The multiplicity of observed difficulties which ensues from initial uncorrected muddle can probably lead to such statements as: 'The striking finding was the diversity of disabilities, and not an underlying pattern common to the group' (Clark 1972). The 'diversity' represents the individual child's developmental pattern interacting with random teaching techniques together with his own phonetic and graphic attempts to reproduce the material.

I hTh a Banin lon he is dafa
he gats my rould and he his z galss bous
From the seabed the bous rna fheul lifts and soufhit.

This is an attempt by a very intelligent nine-year-old boy, without adequate teaching help in rules and regularities, to express the following:

I have a brother-in-law. He is a diver. He gets me sea-urchins and he has three glass bottles from the seabed. The bottles are fossilised and starfish.

In what framework can this language system be taught, then, in order to make it as compatible as possible with the underlying perceptual system of the learner?

6. Diagnosing the difficulty

The first step is simply to be aware of this fundamental developing pattern in many of the children entering school at five years of age; to be aware that it is a perfectly ordinary probability amongst all the other individual differences presented by our child population; that directionally competing sensory, motor and language mechanisms underlie many of the early difficulties in consistent

8

recognition of strings of symbols in exact form. There can be no assumption by teachers that every individual child will automatically acquire this symbolic system. At the spoken language level, auditory confusions will probably have inhibited receptivity to oral sequences of sound, and children with this type of problem tend to be late developers in spoken language. Such maturational lag extends into the written language performance, preventing the necessary competence in relating sound to symbol and perceiving consistent spelling patterns. Recognising and blending sounds, rhyming, learning sequences such as the days of the week, months of the year, seasons, number sequences, etc., will be very difficult for these children. Visual confusion on the other hand will inhibit the consistent appreciation of the *written* forms and present difficulties in establishing learning patterns by the reinforcement of correct responses, that dog is always dog, bed is always bed. Motor ambivalence will inhibit graphic reproduction and writing fluency, preventing the reinforcement which would normally result from constantly perceiving the correct written form before one. Delay in the establishment of unilateral functional areas for language in the brain may inhibit the 'flash' or 'symbolia' needed to encode all these experiences and relate them to meaning. Awareness of these possibilities will enable the teacher to maintain understanding and open attitudes to individual learning needs. Guilt, anxiety, stress and punishment need not enter the learning-teaching relationship.

The second step would seem to be *early diagnosis* of children who are vulnerable in this way. Instruments such as the Aston Index (Newton and Thomson 1974) will enable the teacher, doctor, psychologist or parent to be prepared for these fundamental problems. Some such diagnostic instrument should be available in every beginner class, as well as for appropriate use at later stages. The teacher can then determine the specific difficulty of the individual child. At the present time, first teaching (and often remedial teaching) is a kind of universal scheme for the universal child. Although many reading schemes are published, the teacher is often overwhelmed by the plethora of choice, unsure of the relevance and effectiveness of any particular scheme for the individual child. After basic items to ascertain the level of developing 'intelligence', the Index proceeds to assess the child on a number of items which represent the features of dyslexic difficulties:

Constellations of laterality as described above
Familiar incidence of ambilaterality and difficulties in spelling, reading and fluent writing
The incidence of maturational lag in the family
'At-risk' birth conditions
Socio-cultural opportunities
Visual sequencing ability
Auditory acuity
Auditory sequencing ability
Ability to recite well-known verbal sequences
Knowledge of left/right directions

For the older child:

Performance items of reading, spelling and free writing
A Grapho-motor test
Knowledge of phoneme / grapheme (sound / symbol) correspondences

Scores from these items yield a 'profile' of a child's readiness pattern and individual difficulties. The symptomology can be illustrated by the following case history of a child referred for possible dyslexic-type reading difficulties. This case study is typical of many others seen in clinical practice.

John was referred to the Clinic as a poor reader when he was nine years old. His written work was marked by reversals, mirror-image writing, omissions, random use of capital letters, no punctuation and bizarre spellings. His parents were both professional workers—his father was a University lecturer in mechanical engineering and his mother taught design at the local College of Art. He had a sister eighteen months younger who was doing well at school, except that spelling was still difficult for her. She was left-handed. An older brother was at a Grammar-technical school doing well in science and technical drawing, but finding modern languages and fluent written expression quite difficult.

There had been no apparent difficulties in pregnancy or at birth and milestones had been well within the normal range. Spoken language was, however, late in developing and John was nearly three years old before he started to speak at all fluently. Parents noticed his early ability in spatial/manual tasks such as jigsaws and formboards. John seemed curious, lively and intelligent, and in fact when tested at the Clinic was found to be in the superior range of ability with oral/receptive vocabulary three years in advance of his chronological age. Reading and spelling and written expression, however, were three years retarded. When assessed in psycho-linguistic skills, some difficulties were noted in visual sequential memory, and more severe problems in auditory sequential memory. Sound blending also presented some difficulties.

John had an inconsistent laterality pattern, e.g. he wrote and cut with his right hand, but dealt cards, threaded a needle, threw a ball and screwed a lid with his left. He had not established complete eye dominance, but favoured his left eye in binocular viewing. He was also left-eared. The family pattern of laterality was also mixed: his father was ambidextrous and right-eyed, whereas his mother was right-handed but left-eyed. There was a high incidence of left-handedness in both families. His father had been slow in learning to read but at nine years had made sudden progress and won a place at Grammar School. His mother attended Art School, but was poor at spelling and written fluency. Recently it had been noticed that some secondary emotional difficulties were interacting with John's reading problems and he was withdrawing from any involvement in school activities. At home he was quiet and often near to tears. He was also developing hostile attitudes towards his sister.

'At-risk' birth conditions may also cause maturational delay in the kind of symbolic learning needed for reading and spelling, and can further exacerbate the primary, developmental difficulty. As well as their perceptual confusions, such children show signs of hyper-activity, lack of concentration span, clumsiness and difficulties in motor coordination.

7. Matching the language to the learner

Written language can now be presented to the young learner in a form as compatible as possible with his own pattern of learning. Key points, to be discussed more fully in the next section, are:

Emphasis of the rules and regularities; 85 per cent of the written English language is governed by rules, especially spelling rules.

Relate the rules to the current reading and writing of the individual child—not remote and arbitrary spelling tests given on Friday afternoon (see section 11 on spelling).

Over-teaching and over-learning is essential. Because the perception of direction and order is confused, much more experience of auditory and visual material is needed at every level to enable the child (and the teacher) to reinforce *correct* responses as often as possible and whenever they occur. The 'integrated day' or 'open-plan' teaching is not a good setting therefore in which dyslexic children acquire techniques. The children will not educe or 'catch' the underlying rules unless these are continually reinforced. Attention must be directed in personal teaching to the underlying structures. The teaching of reading and spelling must be a *formal* business; informality being kept for other richness of experience. Creativity and open-ended spontaneity can be expressed in free writing (see later techniques).

Consistency of teaching. One refers again to the overwhelming plethora of printed books and materials available to the teacher. These can be inspected in Teachers' Centres throughout the country, in School Psychological Services, Libraries and in children's book shops. As there are as many individual differences amongst teachers as amongst children, the effective teaching method can very often be the one most compatible with the teacher's own style, provided that visual, auditory and kinaesthetic modes are all employed in the learning situation. Margaret Peters (1972) writes of the success of the 'consistent' teacher, in spite of the particular method used. Some confident selection (or advice for the younger teacher) is needed to resist the passing attractions of new schemes and persuasive arguments of colleagues and salesmen! It is good to know what is available, but effective to choose realistically.

A lively 'integrated' approach, personal to the individual child, combining reading (from a book, not a 'reader', introduced on the first day of teaching and read by the teacher—see Part II) with spelling patterns and free writing. Although the approach is often creative, lively and original for the individual child, published schemes can be a source of great strength. They represent the experience of many workers in the field. They ensure that all aspects and rules are covered and suggest orderly schemes of presentation.

PART 11
Teaching Techniques

8. General guidelines

Most of the following techniques are already in use by many teachers throughout the country. They are brought together in this small volume to serve as basic guidelines for teachers and others who wish to help dyslexic children, and who would welcome some more structured framework in which to work.

First and foremost is the need for individual child-centred teaching. In the case of the beginner-learner this means awareness of general levels of intellectual development, of preparedness for school (socio-emotional factors), of directional, perceptual developmental readiness for symbol-sequencing tasks, and robustness—or otherwise—of individual physiological and neurological development. Factors to be observed include: Is the child under-nourished, lacking energy, hyperactive, or presenting 'at-risk' birth signs? Personality and emotional differences are also important. Is he over-anxious and withdrawn, or conversely aggressive and violent in the playground?

For the older child in a remedial education situation, assessments can be made of his actual performance in school attainment. These scores can be compared to underlying ability ('intelligence') to assess the degree of backwardness or retardation (see section 16). It is also important to note the influence of previous school experience; for example, methods used in teaching, size of classes and other classroom variables.

Knowledge of these factors ensures that an appropriate and compatible programme of learning can be prepared to match the specific needs of the individual child. To enable such profiles of individual children to be drawn, basic assessment instruments should ideally be available to those teachers involved in this kind of work. Effective, realistic teaching can then be planned. This implies relevant training in the necessary techniques.

The personal nature of both first teaching and later remedial teaching must be stressed. In a personal, safe, receptive and understanding teaching environment, the child is free to learn—free from the anxieties and perceived threats which can inhibit the easy exchange of knowledge between teacher and taught. The first teacher would seem to have a very great responsibility, as attitudes to all future learning can be determined at this time. In later remedial work the so-called 'therapeutic' teaching must sometimes redeem a previously feared situation and make it possible for a child to accept and become involved in new learning patterns.

Within this facilitating environment each individual teacher can use his own most effective style. At one time in the Remedial Education Centre mentioned earlier, two schools of thought operated. One was affectionately known as the 'Dudley Zoo' approach and favoured the gradual introduction of the child to academic topics by interesting projects and visits. This approach not only afforded an opportunity for teacher and child to form a trusting relationship through which eventual cognitive studies would begin and flourish, but also provided interesting experiences upon which to base both oral and written language activities. Both aspects, it was thought, would benefit the child's developing self-concept. The other school, however, favoured a more direct approach based on the theory that if reading failure was the presenting difficulty, then immediate steps must be taken at the first session to introduce reading material. A judicious mixture of both approaches was often the result, weighted according to the style of the individual teacher. There were also individual preferences for specific reading schemes. Some remedial teachers (especially males) have been found to favour a logical, formal and structured scheme such as the Royal Road Readers, or the Stott Reading Kits, whilst others would be happy using a free-writing approach to reading, supported by a lively assortment of supplementary reading books and games.

In the clinical situation in which behaviour problems as well as reading failure are being treated, techniques of play therapy are used to enable anxious children to re-live and externalise their fears in fantasy play. Other outlets can be found in the use of the elemental materials of water, sand and clay; painting and finger-painting; lighting fires; canoe-building, climbing and exploring; or the projective devices of the Lowenfield World material, puppetry and psycho-drama. Where unresolved, underlying tensions have produced a 'free-floating' anxiety, inhibiting the child from free involvement in reality (including the task of reading), these catalytic activities often produce a lifting of pressures and consequent opportunities for adjustment and learning.

In the normal school situation there is often the choice between formality and informality. A survey by Goodacre (1967) produced a result showing 35 professed child-centred methodologies against 57 curriculum-centred out of the 100 schools used in the survey. Of the former category, the informality ranges from no scheme at all—the work centred completely around the on-going activity and needs of the children—to eclectic methods combining phonic, look and say, and sentence methods. Today, with the increasing numbers of open-plan schools and integrated days, the situation would appear lively, open to experimentation and providing freedom to select. One refers again to the 'inconsistent' versus 'consistent' teacher and the latter's effectiveness whatever the method used; and to the validity of individual differences in the teaching styles. One would advise each teacher to use his own strengths.

A critical factor in both first and subsequent remedial teaching is the need to present, emphasise and reinforce the *rules and regularities*, the techniques and structure which underlie written language skills. These are essential, whatever the individual style of transmitting them and in whatever school organisation. Reading, spelling and syntax are rule-governed systems, devised by man, and must be taught in a framework of rules.

For safe and confident teaching the teacher must be prepared and well-versed in the knowledge of the underlying structures of language, know where to find books, schemes and reading activities which exemplify these; and be able to present them in interesting, lucid ways to the learner. The place of learning will need the availability of attractive books to cover the range of intellectual age and socio-cultural levels; bookshelves, open storage space, reading games and apparatus; and quiet, well-defined reading areas. The child will need opportunities for free movement to consult reference drawers and shelves; and to have immediate access to lively, colourful wall pictures, book corners and to teaching games. For the teacher who favours a lively, creative and free writing approach, a constant supply of paper, card, wax crayons, felt pens, paints, scissors, stapler, punch, boxes, magazines, etc., will be necessary. Flash cards, spelling cards, rules, reading games and supplementary texts can all be made daily to match the need of the moment. The children themselves will need a continual source of materials for diaries, booklets, notebooks, spelling dictionaries, etc. This method revolves around the child's own experiences which are recorded daily, copied, traced or freely written, read, illustrated and used for selecting relevant spelling rules. This method needs a mature, lively, creative and open attitude on the part of the teacher. If it is to be maximally effective, it must be linked meaningfully and purposefully to a continuing programme of reading, spelling and rule acquisition, which the teacher monitors.

In both first and remedial teaching the need is for flexible and adaptive methods compatible with the specific needs of individual learners. Thus, for example, younger children, or children with neurological diffi- culties, will sometimes need to stand and work in larger media. Long rolls of paper can be pinned to the wall (the back of surplus wallpaper is useful for this purpose) if easels are not available or too space-taking. More sophisti- cated apparatus—over-head projectors, tape recorders, tachistoscope, language-masters, visual aids, even closed- circuit television—are all in use in schools throughout the country. They provide motivational and reinforcement aids in presenting written material and are especially useful in the remedial teaching of older children and where group teaching rather than individual teaching is necess- ary. These 'job aids' are again there to be used on an individually based preference level. Effective teaching is still often accomplished by blackboard and coloured chalk, paper, pencils and books according to the ingenuity, liveliness and ability of individual teachers.

For hyperactive children and those with some form of neurological difficulty it is often necessary (ideally) to teach in a small, quiet place stripped to the bare essentials of desk, book or apparatus, child and teacher, particularly for the more formal part of teaching. When children have difficulty in selective attention, teaching is sometimes effective in short intensive sessions—say ten to fifteen minutes. Such children can be the exception in the need for the very stimulating type of environment. Sometimes the teacher can read a story in a 'shared' situation, with some relevant follow-up activity by the child. Children from socio-economically deprived backgrounds, where perhaps all has been noise and confusion, with no clear 'signal to noise ratio' and no opportunity to attend to any one feature at a time, will also need this help in focusing attention on the matter in hand. It has been discovered that some of the well-meaning 'richness of environment' techniques provided in Head-start programmes in New York schools have lacked a 'perceptual anchor' and failed to initiate true learning involvement. Perhaps some of our open-plan and integrated-days have the same overwhelming features for some children.

Remedial teaching, as first teaching, is set in a personal communication system. The child is free to learn and motivated to do so. Appropriate schemes of work are introduced in a lively positive environment. Paul Widlake reminds us that such teaching can be fun, when released from the anxiety and despair of stereotyped expectation.

9. Guidelines specific to dyslexia

We are concerned with a fundamental fact of early language learning—especially written-language learning.

There is present in the population a high incidence phenomenon—a category of learning difficulty related to the acquisition of sequential symbolic systems. It is a normal feature of development in many children: research suggests that perhaps as many as 28 per cent of the population have this kind of learning pattern to some degree, especially at the early developmental age of five years. It represents an individual difference amongst school children in the manner of perceiving arbitrarily arranged written symbols signifying the meaning of the spoken word. This difference in early perceptual style can be either of genetic origin, present in many members of the same family, or it can be engendered by an 'at-risk' birth situation which delays the normal maturation processes. It appears to be concerned with intrinsic, individual organisations of sensory, motor and language functions of the central nervous system.

These differences in the population have become apparent because of society's demand for universal literacy—the need for every child to begin to learn to read at the early developmental age of five years. Failure to fulfil this expectation has been attributed to various causes since 1870 and the Education Act which set in train the UK educational system.

At first these were of a 'moral' nature—the child who succeeded was 'good', the child who did not was 'bad', 'stupid', or 'lazy'.

Later the environment was seen as the root of the problem—school or home (or both). Then came the era of the 'emotional' causation; the anxiety stresses which prevent the young child from involving in cognitive learning. Running concurrently with these educationally defined causes have been the neurological theories of paediatricians and Medical Officers of Health. However, this decade sees the attempt by many researchers to view the situation in total context—to consider the effects of *all* these predisposing causes in an integrated approach and to understand their effect in relation to the nature of the task—the written-language system itself.

From this it follows that the features of the system which

are incompatible with the young learner's perceptual ability must be recognised. First teaching and remedial teaching can then be devised to match the child's own underlying patterns.

We begin then with an appreciation of this 'interface', or meeting place, between child-learner and language form. Speech forms are represented in written forms by a series of line drawings with invariant features. To the dyslexic observer, however, these so-called invariant features can appear in a random state of flux—to eye, ear and brain. This is thought to be the result of the competing directional systems in the brain itself. So the very first teaching strategies must be concerned with presenting the 'line-drawings' as stable, enduring signals which relate always to specific meanings. The underlying philosophy is one of *perceptual anchors* to prevent the constant shifting of the written trace.

10. Rules and regulations

The first basic rule therefore is that of sound/symbol correspondence. In written language a sound is represented by a specific symbol. A spoken 'A' becomes a written 'a'; 'B' becomes 'b'; 'D' becomes 'd'. Many older children attending for remedial education are found to be lacking in this primary step, which cannot be by-passed at any age. Ingenious methods have been devised for forging the link between the sound-symbol systems. One refers back to the old Beacon method in which mnemonics were introduced into the teaching by means of a continuing story of mother, child and baby. Each family event related to a letter sound/form; e.g. mother was machining a new school skirt for the child; she closed the machine and it looked like 'n'; when it was working it said n-n-n-n-n, etc. The child listens to the telegraph pole on his way home from school. It says l-l-l-l-l—just how it looks. More recently Lynn Wendon has published a pictogram system also based on concrete mnemonics, e.g. the wicked water witch, who sits astride the written 'w'. These mnemonics associate the abstract symbol with the concrete event—a form of transition in representation relating to Piaget's and Bruner's theories of learning—and it fixates the event in a reality situation. Such mnemonic devices transform the abstract 'line-drawings' into meaningful, concrete images which can be associated with meaning and stored in 'schema' form. The teacher also has a link word or phrase to evoke the required response whenever retrieval from memory falters. Other well-used teaching aids are the Edith Norrie Letter Case and the 'Breakthrough to Literacy' apparatus (Helen Arkell of the Dyslexia Institute in London bases a great deal of her teaching on the former). Both of these provide the actual printed letter cards to handle and experience. Games like Scrabble and Lexicon act as reinforcers with older children; lotto or letter-pelmanism with younger children. The activities are followed through by tracing, copying and matching; finding examples on display wall-charts, entering them into personal alphabet books, illustrating, colouring, matching on felt-boards, painting larger versions, etc. As in every stage of teaching the dyslexic child, continual over-reinforcement is necessary.

A related problem is that of upper and lower-case letter muddle. A child may often write and read the names of capital letters but has no understanding of their correspondence to lower-case and sound relationships. This double identification must be *taught*, again in novel and varied ways.

11. Spelling patterns

The next hurdle to be faced is the consistency of spelling patterns. Fortunately there are many permitted digrams and trigrams (i.e. two-letter and three-letter sequences) in the English language. Some of these are composed of vowels, e.g. ee, ea, au, ie: some are consonant strings, e.g. th, ch, st, str, tch, wh, br; some are mixed, e.g. ar, or, end, and, ing. They are all regular structures of the written form of English. Many reading schemes (such as the Gayway, for instance) preface the text by the relevant lists of spelling structures. Gill Cotterell's check-list of spellings is also a useful guide upon which to base the teaching of spelling techniques. A recent publication (Gillham 1974) provides useful lists of common digram and trigram patterns of spelling. The knowledge of these basic constructions can help both the visual and auditory dyslexic (see page 38). The auditory dyslexic especially, with his primary difficulty in retaining sound-series, is faced with a much simpler task if only required to remember two events as opposed to six, e.g. taking the pattern 'ing', which is a very common English letter-string, and learning this as both a sound pattern and a sight pattern, and as a 'chunk' instead of a blend of three separate items. The 'chunk' can then be added to a variety of other spelling chunks, e.g. str, fl, br, cl, go, call, miss, etc. The great difficulty with these children lies in remembering strings of discrete items and retaining them long enough in short-term memory in order that they can be matched in the brain with the stored patterns already there. Thus *meaning* can be ascribed to the 'inkmarks' on the page. It is much more realistic to present spellings in this simplified form. This is based also on sound psychological theory (Miller 1970). This method also helps to prevent the confusion over perceptual features of letters when seen in isolation. The ingenious teacher will be able to combine the spelling patterns in many guises to provide again the necessary over-reinforcement.

Sometimes spelling exercises are used which consist of

discrimination tasks—finding the correct spelling from various other possible combinations, e.g. peice, picee, epcie, piece. The writers have seen blackboards covered with such examples. Such tasks are very confusing to dyslexics, who need to see the *correct* version on every occasion. For them, learning exercises would better consist of repeated copyings and tracings of the correctly spelt word; using it in writing; entering it on card, in colour, into books; reading and repeating it orally; finding it from the pages of old journals, encircling it in colours and copying again into self-made books, etc. Such children also can manage only one or two new spellings on each learning occasion, with reference to spelling family; for example, on one day the emphasis could be on the digrams 'gh' and 'end', on another day it could be on 'th' and 'ar', as they occur in the child's own writing. These discriminatory-type tasks can be used for *testing* perceptual acuity, but in the case of the dyslexic, the writers would warn against their presentation as a remedial teaching technique.

The use of mnemonics is again a useful memory aid. Whenever possible, relate the abstract symbol pattern to a concrete event, e.g. the digram 'gh' can be presented as a pattern brought to Britain by the Norse-men and left in our spelling—'It represents the ghost of the old Vikings, so is silent when inside a word.' The end-letter 'y' can be presented in a rhythmic type of recitation—'happy, funny, silly, jolly; Billy, Betty, Harry, Golly.'

Reciting also helps the technique of blending, which is the next stage in acquiring the competence to recognise new words. One again remembers the old Beacon method of teaching—the five vowels presented on the blackboard in differing colours under which are written lists of example words for the children to 'chant'—'pat-cat-sat-fat-mat: pet-let-get-set-met; pit-lit-sit-fit-bit'. For the child who is acquiring the techniques with ease, this might be a tedious and perhaps an interference task (although a certain amount of reinforcement in the early stages is needed by most), but for dyslexic children it is a source of strength in establishing engrams or memory traces. Young primary-age children usually enjoy these rhythmic repetition recitations anyway and the latency period is well-known for its receptivity to rule and regularities—learning at these basic simple levels. (It is a much more difficult task for a retarded adolescent boy, for instance, to learn number tables.) As Stockhausen has said: 'Rhythm is order in sound.' As perceiving order is the difficulty for the dyslexic child, rhythm can provide another form of perceptual anchor.

Every device for novel representations of the spelling rules must be sought. The four stages are:

recognition
relating sound to symbols
re-call
use in free writing.

For the first three of these stages, the copying/tracing techniques can again be used: entering spellings into self-made dictionaries, onto card (stacked in toast-racks) or into simple file-index systems for older children; into note-books of different sizes and shapes (long, thin, vertical or lengthwise; square; fan-shaped, etc.). Professor Miles' useful little book *On helping the dyslexic child* provides detailed teaching aids on these phonic techniques. One other key point is to avoid presenting similar shapes simultaneously; not 'b' and 'd' or 'ea' and 'ee' on the same day. Use contrast shapes for aiding discrimination.

12. Thought units
Another instance of 'chunking' as a form of perceptual

anchor is in the actual planning of the amount of text per line and the arrangement of line upon page. This applies both to reading and to free writing. First readers would ideally be written with a small amount of text per page, arranged in 'thought units', i.e. meaningful, short combinations of words within the span of recognition. Organising the material in this way helps to prevent the possibility of confused directional attack. This prevents the 'barking at print' (word-by-word) type of performance, encourages directional fluency and minimises regressive eye movements—which in turn speeds up the actual reading time. There are motivational advantages also, in that the child is able to grasp the meaning of what he reads and can enjoy the story context. When the teacher is helping in the first free-writing situation, the 'thought unit' organisation can be used when writing down the first copy of the child's orally-produced story. Each line of written story can consist of two, three or four words only, which enclose in themselves a meaningful phrase. When the child is able to make his own stories, he can be encouraged at first to use this 'chunking' strategy.

13. Presentation

Spellings should all be related to either the reading book or the child's own writing. Attempts to learn arbitrary lists of spellings as separate drills unrelated to context usually meet with little lasting success, and indeed form a kind of negative conditioning to failure. This in turn blocks the child emotionally from successful learning even when he might be ready at eight or nine years to perceive the arbitrary strings in consistent form. Spelling patterns, or spelling families, which generalise from the specific image in the child's own writing, can however be presented as rules to be learnt. Adolescents or older adults often need reassuring and therapeutic modes of teaching spelling and writing. As the confused perceptual difficulty seems part of a maturational lag process, many people *could* grasp the rules with comparative ease at later stages. But the association with early, often humiliating failure can prevent learning and recognition even when readiness stages are reached. Many different modes of presenting spellings can be found in the books of A. E. Tansley, in the Ladybird series, in Breakthrough to Literacy, Royal Road Readers, Stott's Kits, Stillman & Gillingham, Gill Cotterell's publication *Diagnosis in the Classroom;* and indeed many other schemes may be found in Teachers' Centres and libraries. Although many creative teachers devise their own systems, it is useful sometimes to refer to authorities and experts in the field. It ensures comprehensive coverage of rules and helps in organising material in meaningful sequence.

14. Reading

We have been discussing some basic techniques for perceiving and interpreting the underlying rules and techniques of written language. A major problem for the dyslexic, however, lies in getting pleasure and information from the task of reading itself. So books must be presented as desirable, interesting, exciting or amusing things. The writers would themselves introduce books from the very first day, even in the first learning situation. Special care must be taken in selection: the book must be attractive, appropriate to age and interest, short and well illustrated. Although it is invidious to mention any one scheme from the plethora of available material, perhaps one could draw attention to the new Holt-Bond Readers which are now being used in so many American schools. These were especially written and designed by a team of experts and provide perhaps an extra motivating power for the dyslexic child—something special, glossy and looking rather like presents! On the first occasion the teacher simply reads aloud a page or two of story—either in a one-to-one relationship with the learner or in a very small group situation—and follows with a short discussion, making reference to the story's characters and illustrations, etc. The children could then make a corresponding picture under which the teacher writes a small legend. This could be the beginning of a series of self-made books by the child. Eventually he would take part in the story reading, following the text as the teacher reads. He could then whisper the story as she reads it again—then he reads while she whispers—or she pauses now and then, hoping for the child to supply the next word. It is sometimes useful to have two book-markers (simply made from card, about 5×2 inches and decorated by crayon, etc.). One marker tracks the path across the page, under the line of text from left to right; the other points the way *down* the page, line by line and held by the left hand. These two 'job-aids' stabilise direction and place on the page (often part of the dyslexic's difficulty) and as such become yet another form of perceptual anchor. Some children, and especially older children, like to keep a record of all the books they read by noting them on the book-marker.

If reading is introduced in this pleasant, non-anxious, non-punitive way there is a better chance of fostering receptive attitudes in the child, so often a problem because of the difficult nature of the task and the enormous amount of disciplined hard work the dyslexic child must invest in it. Children who are still failing after the age of eight develop very powerful avoidance mechanisms and it is often one of the first tasks of the remedial teacher to re-kindle interest and motivation.

Many different books are needed for each level of progress, so numerous readers of equivalent difficulty will be necessary at each 'plateau'. No attempts must be made at a 'syllabus' or at reaching a certain goal by any one time. One observes and follows the child, consolidating each achievement, however small. It is important to mention here that a child with dyslexic difficulties will regress to earlier levels, or lose the skill temporarily, if under any severe stress. Such stress might have its origins in sickening for some illness, becoming emotionally blocked by a transient family anxiety or troubled by some event in school itself. Children disabled by enduring socio-cultural deprivation will be even more vulnerable to stress. The teacher needs to be aware of these vulnerabilities and not become personally anxious or despairing. On difficult days the teacher should continue the story-reading, the oral reinforcement, the reading games, etc., but should not expect dramatic progress.

The selection of appropriate books is important. Content should be within the reader's apprehension span and also sufficiently related to familiar events to make sense. Efforts have been made by authors such as Allen Pullen and Cyril Rapstock (in their 'Inner Ring' series) and Leila Berg's 'Nippers' to present very familiar incidents of life to children in less favoured socio-economic environments. To the present writers these books would seem to be helpful in the initial stages of remedial education, presenting the 'known', but should also lead on to topics of wider interest: adventure, fantasy, simple versions of well-known folk tales and children's classics—on to the unknown, in fact, and the extension of experience which underlies one important facet of education. The teacher's task is to determine what is appropriate at any given time. One of the present writers once attempted to present *The Secret Garden* to an 'opportunity' class of adolescent girls in a fairly deprived industrial city, at a very early stage in the remedial programme. The conceptual 'leap' was too great at that time and the book was badly received. Other, more familiar stories should have been presented first.

Although not common practice at the present time, one still sees older boys reading the Infants-type readers. As a general rule this is a bad situation—for motivational and for 'self-concept' reasons as well as for inadequate interest level. The writers have known of instances, however, when really resistive boys of twelve and thirteen years have chosen some very simple early books on which to carry them over the threshold of reading. One such case is reported in *Remedial Education* (Vol. 6, No. 3, Nov. 1971). The books were *chosen*, however, not presented arbitrarily by the teacher as part of the reading programme. There are many simplified versions now available of books based on ideas compatible with older children's chronological and social levels.

Many older children in the writers' clinical experience have learned to read from books on hobbies, crafts, technical subjects and instruction manuals. One group of four thirteen-year-olds constructed a crystal radio from a simplified instruction manual. The subsequent involvement in many forms of written language based on this activity established firm beginnings of reading skills. One non-reader (girl) of eleven years began by using fashion design magazines, making a simple garment and interpreting the instructions in written form. Another boy of nine was found to have a passionate interest in guns. As we were in the notable gun-makers city of Birmingham, a visit to a manufacturer was arranged, literature collected and the whole event written up in diary form. Again, we were over the threshold of recognition and insight. Children's hobbies can all be used in the service of acquiring the written word—fishing, photography, football, television, skin-diving, steam-engines, aircraft, vintage comedy films, pop stars, collecting matchbox jokes, etc., have all been the means of 'crossing the threshold'.

15. The writing approach to reading

Previous sections have been concerned with the techniques of reading and spelling. This section will attempt to set these techniques in a first or remedial-teaching setting; to present guidelines on the *logistics* of teaching in fact. Referring back to individual styles of teaching and the benefits of consistent teaching, one can only make suggestions related to personal preference. Other, perhaps more formal routines, would be equally effective if carried out by enthusiasts and believers in differing creeds.

For the present writers, then, the 'writing approach to reading' combines the 'best of all worlds' when helping the dyslexic child. Ideally in a one-to-one relationship between child and teacher, the session can last from ten minutes (for the hyperactive child) to twenty minutes (beginner-learner) to sixty minutes in a remedial situation with an older child, one or two such sessions per day. Efforts are often concentrated on *reading* only, on the grounds that once this skill is acquired, writing and spelling will follow. In fact reading is a different skill from writing. It is a kind of 'pattern' recognition, directly linked to a template, an existing given form. Writing, however, like spelling, must be organised from internal sources with no perceptual cues and guides. It must therefore be a learning process concomitant with reading if skills are to develop.

The session will begin with a piece of creative writing. For the beginner-learner (of any age) this will start as a spoken account by the child of some event of topical interest—'Well, what has happened today then?'—from news of pets, clubs, friendships; funny, sad, beautiful, ugly, interesting, frightening, happy 'things'; dreams, make-believe, grumbles, events from the cat stuck in the tree to the broken 'fridge' will all provide a medium of communication to be conveyed to the page.

The spoken account is written by the teacher, preferably

in self-made books, plain pages, say eight inches by five, stapled together in cardboard covers decorated by the child. A realistically short passage is chosen initially (one sentence for very young, or very disabled older children) and is traced and copied; re-read by teacher and child, then illustrated; then read again. (Books made entirely from tracing paper are attractive in themselves, if bound in cardboard covers.) Parents attending a diagnostic and advisory clinic at Aston are shown a variety of 'free writing' books which can be bought commercially. Each one has some novelty feature to capture the interest of the reluctant learner. For example, one is a very large, long book, the cover being illustrated by a picture of an elephant and the words 'Elephants never forget'. The pages are divided into three framed areas which serve for first copy, corrected copy and spelling pattern corrections. Autograph books can be adaped as story books and are often the ideal size for the first attempt at story writing—two or three sentences only on a page, with an appropriate picture on the facing page. Older boys are motivated to write in enlarged business-type desk diaries, and even enjoy writing a daily account of their activities in such form. The commercial books serve as a model, but of course similar books can be made to supplement these from the materials previously mentioned.

For the young beginner-learner a 'sound' can be isolated, initally perhaps the letter 'a' from the written text, attention drawn to the correspondence with graphic form, some mnemonic system used and finally the letter entered into another, smaller self-made book (perhaps directory-typewith alphabetic edges, or long and thin, etc.) and copied several times, in many colours say. Perhaps the word containing the sound could be made from Breakthrough letters or Edith Norrie letter case and the letter on the corresponding wall-chart pointed out.

The rest of the session is used for reading from a book, especially selected on this occasion by the teacher as appropriate to age, interest and social level of the learner. The story is read completely by the teacher. As sessions continue, however, the techniques of whispering, etc., described earlier, can be introduced until finally the child is recognising words spontaneously and joining in the reading task.

This can be the basic format and can be modified, enlarged and varied by the addition of any special experience in spelling (as in section 11); writing, tracing, writing-patterns (the Marion Richardson writing-patterns still provide valuable kinaesthetic experience in graphic direction and order); experiencing letters in different textures, e.g. velvet and sand-paper, again for kinaesthetic reinforcement; a continuing lively use of spoken language as the basis for creative writing; the use of overhead projectors for spelling and syntax rules for small groups of older children; or individual work with teaching-machines, again to provide reinforcement for rules learnt. Lyn Lewis, Head of the Remedial Department of Millfield School, uses many technological devices to very good effect in teaching older children in his department. Writing of letters at appropriate times; accounts of projects, visits and interesting events in school and society; and finally books themselves, presented in a continuity of activity as part of the freely chosen experience, all strengthen the child's power to accomplish the desired task.

This global approach to written language acquisition, as well as relating all aspects in one meaningful schema, fulfils the criteria of a *VAK* approach, as introduced by Samuel Orton nearly thirty years ago. This combined visual, auditory and kinaesthetic approach to reading and writing is still used extensively in parts of America, especially by Sally Childs in Dallas, and in the UK by Agnes Wolfe of the Bath Institute of Dyslexia. The present writers use the mnemonic 'W, double r' to represent the teaching sequence—writing, rule, reading!

16. Guide to grouping

Much stress is laid in both first and remedial education on individual, child-centred work and in many cases a start to real learning is best made in such a facilitating one-to-one relationship. There are, however, situations in which group teaching is the only possible setting. The heavy demands of specialist teaching in the clinic situation sometimes make it necessary for a child to begin in a one-to-one situation, but once over the 'threshold to learning', he joins a small group for further work. Sometimes this can even be of benefit to an anxious or solitary child in providing the first steps in adapting to the larger group situation of school. In a well-matched group, also, children can help each other.

Remedial education in the school situation generally places emphasis on group rather than individual teaching for obvious reasons, although provision is made in some places for individual tuition from visiting remedial teachers, or from a specialist teacher who is a staff member of the school. Where group teaching is necessary, however, it is of vital importance to plan the groups with certain criteria in mind.

Supposing, for instance, one were providing 'opportunity rooms' for children with learning difficulties in secondary schools. As a first step, a survey of the ability and attainment of all new entrants could be made; and on the results of such measures children would be allocated to groups for appropriate teaching. In a large school this could mean various sets for English or Arithmetic, including the 'special opportunity' sets for children who appeared to be in one of the following groups:

1. Those children whose underlying general ability would appear to be in the average or above-average range, but who were seriously retarded in written language skills (or mathematics).
2. Those children who would fall into the category of slow learning generally and who were failing in school attainments as part of this type of developmental pattern.

The former category is usually referred to as 'retardation', measured by discrepancy from mental age; whereas the latter category is described as backwardness, and poor performance is related to chronological age. It would seem necessary for effective remedial teaching to separate out these two categories, as the needs of children belonging to one or the other are very different. The 'retardates' are often able to devise and use their own strategies to acquire and remember the rules; to respond more quickly to suggestion and precept; to utilise a lively flow of ideas and oral fluency upon which to base their written work; to achieve progress by sudden insights; to use context clues in reading; to benefit by a lively 'w, double r' approach; to respond to a mature use of oral language in the early stage of development, probably on the basis of language exchange with the teacher; to involve themselves in many projects upon which written language can be based; and to need a more socially-mature type of reading material. In general, if good teaching is available, these intelligent but specifically retarded children will proceed more quickly and more independently than the 'slow-learners.'

The latter will need very much material of the same level at each stage. Each step, stage, sound/symbol correspondence, spelling pattern, word-picture, page of text, etc., will need to be presented in many guises and reinforced with many support activities. The language used in transmitting the learning will need to be paced appropriately and match the child's own basic schema. Much repetition will be necessary. The child's own ideas can still be exploited, but more help, encouragement and 'props' provided to elicit the responses. A strategy of continuing question-and-answer is often an effective way of utilising language at a relevant level. In general, also, these children will need a different array of books from which to choose.

One must be aware, however, of the dangers of making arbitrary judgments on results of tests. Cases have come to the writers' attention of children of eight, ten or even fourteen years, who have been assessed as 'educationally sub-normal' at an early stage of development, probably on the basis of their language difficulty, and who have then been regarded as slow-learners until some perceptive teacher has recognised their true potential (adult dyslexics have also reported this state of affairs). This has been masked by a specific developmental lag in perception of the dyslexic kind. Teaching in a small group will enable the teacher to perceive the true nature of the learning difficulty.

One of the writers used the above survey method, for appropriate allocation to groups, when establishing 'opportunity' groups in secondary schools in a Midlands industrial town. The method was helped by the fact that each year was set for basic subjects, so that when children joined their English or Mathematics set, the remedial groups joined their 'opportunity' classes, returning to their all-ability groups for other topics.

In considering the logistics of planning remedial help within each school, it would seem that the needs of the primary school would differ from the secondary stage.

The primary school could perhaps be served by a specialist remedial teacher who can advise other teachers as well as taking small groups and individual children herself, and by keeping a 'remedial' room stocked with equipment and library facilities to which all staff could have access when necessary. At the secondary stage, it would seem effective to appoint 'counsellors', especially trained in child psychology and remedial method. Children with any anxiety or learning problem could be referred to such specialists and problems often solved in a transient situation. Reading problems would be only one (albeit an important one) category of difficulty to help in the ordinary day-to-day running of the school. A remedial language department would be one of the normal school facilities. Such departments do in fact exist. The training of specialists in all the individual patterns of development and appropriate methods of treatment would seem to be an urgent priority, especially in the large urban schools. The dyslexic problem is a key issue in this context, relating as it does to the 'coinage' of secondary education, which is the written language system of the culture.

17. Visual, auditory and graphic aspects of dyslexia

The dyslexic language difficulty can be in any one sensory mechanism or in any combination. Children who have directional confusion in auditory interpretation often present the greatest problems to the teacher, especially in spelling and expressive writing. As they often do not hear the signal in arbitrarily ordered form, spellings can be bizarre—e.g. 'tilf' can represent 'elephant'; 'agt' is 'gate'. If there is an underlying difficulty of temporal ordering, blending phonemes into morphemes, into words, phrases, sentences, etc., in the desired sequence and direction, retrieval from memory of arbitrary patterns is very difficult. These children need the massive over-learning and over-teaching of spelling rules and regularities, phoneme/grapheme correspondences and many varied opportunities for presenting them. For these children rhymes, rhythms (both spoken and tympanic), songs, drama and many verbal exchanges will also be helpful in establishing organised order.

The visual dyslexic often has the mirror-image syndrome; was/saw; on/no; girl/gril; brid/bird; form/from; god/dog. He will sometimes scan from right to left, lose his place on the page, have regressive eye-movements which slow down performance; mis-place words in reading. (Both auditory and visual dyslexic types seem to miss commas, full stops, capital letters, etc., and need to re-read the text for meaning as the first reading is confined to a mastery of techniques.) Brightly coloured margins down the left hand side of pages will be perceptual anchors; use of two markers referred to earlier; quick recognition games, such as snap, lotto, flash cards, etc.; matching, over-learning of the digram and trigram, spelling patterns and the use of chunking—all these activities will supplement the daily reading and free-writing activities. A useful new publication to help with perceptual ordering is by Juliet Reeve and Jean Jackson and is called *Look*.

The 'dysgraphia' problem is helped by all the above techniques, but especially by tracing, writing patterns, 'texture' exercises, Fernald (1943) techniques and daily experience of written expression. It might be helpful to give such children the perceptual anchors of lines across the page, spaced at half an inch intervals at first, between which to write. For neurological, motor problems, specially supported pens and pencils can be used. The writers were shown an ingenious example of these, devised by Kathleen Hickey of the Guildford Institute of Dyslexia.

Sometimes a child, especially at the young developmental age of first learning, can be handicapped in all these sensory and motor mechanisms, or in two of them. A careful, patient, teaching programme needs instituting from the first day, combining relevant techniques from all methods.

PART 111

Other Points of Interest

Various recurring features of dyslexia have been observed clinically over the past years. These are now listed to serve as guide lines for treatment and advice to others involved in helping and teaching children and adults with this primary language difficulty.

18. Some notes on the change-over from left to righthand
It frequently happens that teachers and parents are faced with the problem of a left-handed child starting school in a 'right-handed' world. Because the written forms of language scan from left to right in English-speaking (and many other) countries, it would seem that the left-handed child is at a disadvantage in acquiring this one-directional skill. He will have a motor tendency in the first place to write from right to left on the page. Then, when writing in the *required* direction, a left-handed child will be obscuring his line of text as he writes, thus depriving him of some continuity of experience.

There will also be conflicts of direction, both perceptual and motor, and a tendency to regress therefore, or make non-fluent movements, or inconsistencies in the slope of writing. Sometimes a left-handed child is also left-eyed and will be visually scanning the material from right to left. Consequently, spelling patterns become disturbed as well as the arrangement of words in a sentence; in fact he will have difficulties with fluency of reading and writing in general. Because of these ambiguities in direction, work is slowed down and undue time has to be taken to complete the ordinary demands of prose writing.

What advice could be given therefore to help a child with these left-sided tendencies in a right-sided world?

It is very difficult to generalise about modifying the left/right motor/directional biases of each individual child, as each one has a different underlying constellation of laterality ('sidedness'). One must observe very closely the *total* behaviour of the child as he uses hand, eye and foot for all the activities of the day. If the left hand is used continually for all the finer movements of writing, cutting (scissors), painting, spoon, knife, etc., it would appear that there is a strong organisational (internal) preference for 'leftness' in motor tasks. In this case one would not seek to change to right-handed mode. If, however, the child uses either hand at random both for fine and gross movements and is having severe directional problems in writing and reading, a programme of remedial help could be devised starting from a physiological level, which could mean emphasising *right*-handed motor activitity in a left/right direction. These children seem to be rare, however, amongst the total population of ambilateral people (many of whom, although not seeming to have established a hand or eye dominance, in the final analysis prefer one side or the other for motor movements).

Because handedness is a part of an underlying complex organisation in the brain, the advice seems to be, in the main, not to change a child except in the rare circumstances mentioned above (especially over the age of 5), but to give him strategies within his own patterning for dealing with the demands of school learning, etc. These would include, of course, many left to right-type patternings, tracings, always starting from a brightly coloured margin on the left (helping the child to notice differences in direction, especially in letters, words, sentences, etc.) and using a book marker, both for drawing along the line as one reads, and also for moving down the page on the left indicating the beginning of each line of text. It is a continual process of over-teaching in which over-learning is needed to enable the child to adapt to the desired directional/sequential system when he himself would perhaps acquire more easily a spatial or iconic one. One can reinforce directional awareness in other activities, e.g. arrangement of tools, pencils, play equipment, table placings and everyday objects of life.

Needless to say, one gives the child many opportunities to succeed in his own skills of painting, modelling, kit-making, etc., to achieve satisfactory psychic development as well as specific language-orientated creative writing, spelling pattern learning and 'reading for fun.'

19. Changes of neurological patterning

Where a child has been born at risk, remedial programmes of motor coordination can be devised. When advised by the Specialist these can be beneficial, but cannot in themselves provide remediation in reading. A well constructed programme of learning is still necessary.

The ontogenetic progress of each child follows very individual growth patterns (Tanner and Inhelder 1957). It would seem to the writers, in the present state of knowledge, inadvisable to try and change the course of any one mechanism. Instead, treatment must be within the language presentation itself, on the principle of 'perceptual anchors' as described in the text; enabling the child to perceive and practise direction within his own underlying organisation.

20. Higher education

Intelligent students with dyslexic-type language difficulties have been found to succeed at CSE and GCE examinations in geography, geology, biology, engineering drawing, technical drawing, pharmacy, art, geometry and zoology in schools where understanding and support are given to the deficiencies in reading and written English.

The common factor in all these topics seems to be the spatial, symmetrical, balanced nature of the skill involved, in contrast to the uni-directional and arbitrary nature of symbolic systems. The case histories of many of these students reveal both genetic and occupational relationships in other members of the families, e.g. successful careers in the adult members of both maternal and paternal families in civil engineering, surgery, dental surgery, draughtsmanship, tailoring, design, athletics, architecture and art, together with left-handedness, left-eyedness and ambilaterality.

Common features of referral in students presenting with dyslexic difficulties are:

1. Slow reading, marked by regressive eye-movements hindering fluent left-right directional scanning of the written text and resulting in repeated attempts to read one line, as meaning gets lost in the difficulty over techniques. This is particularly frustrating where 'skimming' is needed for the great amount of literature to be served in higher education.
2. Spelling errors, giving a false impression of retarded scholarship and also slowing down rate of work output because of constant checking.

3. Lack of fluency in writing essays, reports, projects, etc. Again the difficulties are those of time-taking and of giving a false impression of oral and comprehension ability.

One sometimes gets a piece of writing more typical of an eight-year-old from a very able engineering and physics student. This incompatibility between thinking power and effective problem-solving on the one hand and immature spelling and writing on the other is a source of great frustration to the able student. Even worse, it can result in a potentially very able student being refused entry to a higher education course.

Individual differences in thinking styles, especially symbolic *vis-à-vis* spatial, is no new idea. Renowned psychologists such as Cyril Burt and Philip Vernon in the UK, and J. P. Guilford in America, have written at length about such differences in man's abilities. McFarlane-Smith has spent over thirty years studying the phenomenon of spatial ability.

Of direct interest to the educationist is the use of these insights in an applied manner, i.e. a compatibility of skill learning with the potential of the learner. Not only is human fulfilment and happiness at risk, but also the effective contribution to society's needs of the people with such abilities.

Once again the urgency of early diagnosis must be reiterated. This may prevent emotional distress, permanent sense of failure, breakdown in adulthood, feelings of worthlessness, and delinquency and crime in less supported members of community. This highlights the need for early diagnostic cues such as are outlined in the Aston Index.

Written language forms the basis of all formal education, and it is therefore necessary that children acquire written language skills if they are to pass successfully through the system. This means that the teacher must be able to maximise each child's potential, despite particular difficulties he or she may have.

The difficulties described in this book may reflect different etiologies; these include the genetic and familial aspects, which may represent a 'pure' developmental dyslexia, as well as 'at risk' birth situations which may minimally affect cognitive or perceptual functions. Another important point is the high proportion of boys to be found in this category of learning difficulty, which could be related to genetic factors.

Dyslexia is often called a 'middle-class' phenomenon; this myth reflects the vocal and well informed section of the community who can express their children's anxieties and who speak for *all* parents, and not the actual category of learning difficulty, which occurs in all *socio-economic levels*. This specific difficulty in written language is of course more marked in able children and will tend to be masked in less intelligent and deprived children (because these other difficulties manifest themselves, and therefore teachers do not look for any other possible added situation).

21. Helping the dyslexic to help himself

This section applies equally to the adult dyslexic and to the child. Failure to read, write and spell can produce a general feeling of incompetency in all matters relating to books or written information of any kind. There is a subsequent reluctance therefore to use any of the support systems provided by educational services and society in general, if these are language-based. Part of the teaching must be directed therefore to instruction on the use of libraries, reference shelves, reference books, manuals and written procedures. Attention must be drawn to notices, labels, announcements and instructions in the surrounding environment. If early teaching begins in this supported situation, receptive habits to interpreting and retrieving such information will be established.

22. Operant conditioning

At the time of writing, research into operant-conditioning approaches to remediation are being investigated; shaping behaviour by reinforcing schedules of learning in the desired directions. This is task-oriented learning and scientifically planned. It is a method based on Dr Skinner's work and seems to have found some application to treating behaviour disorders in children. Its relevance to the teaching of dyslexic children could be investigated. Such methods are intended as auxiliary to more conventional ones, not to replace the link between the teacher and the taught. If we consider the learning situation to be a communication system in which knowledge and skill is transmitted in psycho-social manner, we must look at the person-oriented aspects of acquiring skills also. In this context, behaviourists' theory would perhaps be acceptable to people at present threatened by its mechanistic approach.

PART IV

Recapitulation

Societies in which universal literacy is sought are faced with a special educational problem in the very earliest stages. A considerable number of children will arrive at school to take part in formal symbolic learning without having reached an appropriate developmental stage of consistent sensory and motor mechanisms. A consistent stage of development is necessary to perceive the arbitrarily ordered sequences of a written alphabet. There will be many individual differences in the readiness to acquire this alphabetic system. The differences can relate to both genetic, constitutional factors, or to vulnerabilities caused by at-risk birth situations. But they all represent a *primary* intrinsic category of learning potential. The category is described in this monograph— as in many countries throughout the world—as dyslexia, or dyslexic-type language difficulty. The problem of learning can be exacerbated by such secondary factors as emotional stresses, intellectual deficit, socio-cultural deprivations, over-large classes, unsuitable teaching methods and inadequately prepared teachers, etc. These are added stresses to the primary difficulty. The dyslexic category of written-language difficulty, however, can be independent of intelligence, socio-economic opportunity or emotional stress.

Early diagnosis is necessary in order to establish appropriate teaching programmes and to prevent social, emotional and intellectual failure. Teachers must be prepared and trained therefore in necessary diagnostic techniques.

After diagnosis, teaching schemes compatible with each child's developmental readiness can be planned. It is suggested that an underlying philosophy of *perceptual anchors* is adopted. Language is presented as a system of rules, orders and regularities which can be reinforced by concrete mediational strategies and relevant mnemonics. The teaching environment matches the individual level and need. Special attention is paid to motivational aspects, since the dyslexic person needs to work very hard and 'over-learn' in order to acquire the system.

Liveliness, creativity, constant efforts to maintain interest, 'global' involvement by the child, a writing approach to reading, etc., are all suggested as key factors in teaching. The support of published schemes is acknowledged.

In all methods of presentation, however, individual teaching styles and the value of consistent, stable approaches of instruction are recognised. The effectiveness of any teaching method would seem to be in its *interpretation* in relation to the realistic need of the learner.

Also recognised are the specific abilities of many dyslexic persons and recommendations are made for personal fulfilment and voational guidance.

Having demanded the acquisition of written language skills, society is responsible for providing the means of transmitting them effectively to each of its individual members.

When this is finally achieved, there will be no 'dyslexia'.

Useful Reading Schemes

Many successful schemes of work are in progress in School Remedial Teaching Services throughout the country. A notable example is the Birmingham Service headed by David Fudge. Detailed accounts of four such services are available for inspection in the Developmental Language Study Centre of Aston University and have been duplicated by kind permission of the Authors. These are:

BEAZLEY, J. County Council of Essex.
FISH, E. Basildon Committee for Education, Essex.
FOSKETT, J. Cornwall Education Committee.
KELLY, G., THOMPSON, G. Child Psychological Service, West Bromwich.

Many reading schemes have been mentioned in the text; these and others can be inspected at local libraries, Teachers' Centres, Child Guidance Clinics, School Psychological Services, etc.

A number of these reading schemes are also mentioned in Gillham (1974).

Glossary

Cerebral dominance — term originally used by neurologists to describe the hemisphere of the brain which processes language.

Dysgraphia — disturbance in the visuo-motor system, resulting in extreme difficulty with production of the written form.

Etiology — underlying causation of difficulty.

Hyperactivity — disorder affecting arousal mechanisms, resulting in difficulties in inhibiting inappropriate activity (e.g. movement, attention).

Iconic — appertaining to the concrete or image in the environment (gk. — icon).

Kinaesthetic — appertaining to muscle sense and movement, by which weight, motion and position are perceived.

Laterality — sidedness (left/right), mainly relating to sensory (eye, ear) and motor (hand/foot) mechanisms, or at another level to left and right hemispheres of the brain involved in different functions.

Modality — organisation of sensation by different organs: e.g. visual modality, information from the eyes; auditory modality, information from ears.

Neurological — relating to structure and function in the central nervous system.

Sound blending — skill of putting sounds together to make words, e.g. *c* (hard sound) - *a* - *t* makes *cat*.

Symbolia — global identification of a word as a whole, as a symbolic entity related to meaning.

Tachistoscope — apparatus for flashing stimuli at controlled time intervals or light intensities.

References

ANNETT, M. (1963) 'A model of the inheritance of handedness and cerebral dominance.' *Nature*, *204*, 59–60.

BINET, A. and SIMON, T. (1905) 'Methodes nouvelles, pour le diagnostic du niveau intellectual des anormaux.' *L'Annee psychologique*, Vol 2.

BRUNER, J. S. (1964) 'The course of cognitive growth.' *Amer Psychol.*, *19*, 1–19.

BURT, C. (1937) *The Backward Child*. London: University of London Press.

CATTY, N. (1933) *Modern Education of Younger Children*. London: Methuen.

CLARK, M. (1972) Quoted in *Children with Specific Reading Difficulties*. D.E.S. publication. London: H.M.S.O.

COLLINS, J. E. (1967) *The Effects of Remedial Education*. Institute Monographs on Education, University of Birmingham.

COTTERELL, G. (1973) *Diagnosis in the Classroom*. Reading Centre, University of Reading.

CRITCHLEY, M. (1970) *The Dyslexic Child*. London: Heinemann.

FERNALD, G. M. (1943) *Remedial Techniques in Basic School Subjects*. New York: McGraw-Hill.

GATES, A. I. and BOND, G. L. (1936 'Reading Readiness, a study of factors determining success and failure in beginning reading.' *Teach. Coll. Rec. 37*, 679–85.

GIBSON, E. J. (1965) 'Learning to read.' *Science, 148*, 3673, 1066–72.

GILLHAM, W. E. C. (1974) *Teaching a Child to Read.* London: University of London Press.

GOODACRE, E. J. (1967) *Reading in Infant Classes.* Slough: N.F.E.R.

HALLGREN, B. (1950) 'Specific dyslexia: a clinical and genetic study.' *Acta Psychiat. Neurol. Scand. Suppl. 65.*

KAWI, A. A. and PASAMANICK, B. (1959) *Prenatal and Paranatal Factors in the Development of Childhood Reading Disorders.* Monograph of the Society for Research into Child Development, Lafayette.

MILES, T. (1970) *On Helping the Dyslexic Child.* London: Methuen Educational.

MILLER, G. A. (1970) 'The magical number seven.' In *The Psychology of Communication.* Harmondsworth: Penguin.

NEWTON, M. (1968) *A Neuro-psychological Investigation into Dyslexia.* A. P. Report no. 25, University of Aston in Birmingham.

NEWTON, M. (1974) 'Towards diagnosis of dyslexia.' Paper given at the conference of the British Dyslexia Association, Churchill College, Cambridge, September 1974.

NEWTON, M. and THOMSON, M. (1974) '*Towards* diagnosis of dyslexic difficulties.' *Dyslexia Review, 11.*

ORTON, S. T. (1937) *Reading, Writing and Speech Problems in Children.* London: Chapman and Hall.

PETERS, M. (1972) 'The teaching of spelling.' Paper in the Proceedings of the Specific Learning Disabilities course, College of Education, Madeley, Staffs.

PRINGLE, M. L. K. (1952) *The Remedial Education Centre, University of Birmingham*. Birmingham: Institute of Education.

REEVE, J. and JACKSON, J. (1972) *Look*. London: Macmillan.

SCHONELL, F. (1942) *Backwardness in the Basic Subjects*. Oliver and Boyd.

TANNER, J. and INHELDER, B. (eds.) (1957) *Discussions on Child Development; a Consideration of the Biological, Psychological and Cultural Approaches to Understanding Human Development and Behaviour*. London: Tavistock.

TIZARD, J. (1972) *Children with Specific Reading Difficulties*. D.E.S. publication. London: H.M.S.O.

VERNON, M. D. (1957) *Backwardness in Reading*. Cambridge: Cambridge University Press.

ZANGWILL, O. and BLAKEMORE, C. (1972) 'Dyslexia: reversal of eye movements during reading.' *J. Neuropsychol.*, *10*, 371-3.

Other Source Books on Background Material

BAKKER, D. and SATZ, P. (1970) *Specific Reading Disability*. Rotterdam: Rotterdam University Press.

BANNATYNE, A. (1971)*Language, Reading and Learning Disabilities*. Springfield, Illinois: Charles C. Thomas.

FRANKLIN, A. W. and NAIDOO, S. (Eds.) (1970) *Assessment and Teaching of Dyslexic Children*. I.C.A.A.

HEPWORTH, T. S. (1971) *Dyslexia: The Problems of Reading Retardation*. Sydney: Angus and Robertson.

JORDAN (1972) *Dyslexia in the Classroom*. New York: C. Merrill Co.

KEENEY, A. and KEENEY, V. (1968) (Eds.) *Dyslexia Diagnosis and Treatment of Reading Disorders*. New York: C. V. Mosby and Co.

KLASEN, E. (1972) *The Syndrome of Specific Dyslexia*. Lancaster: Medical and Technical Publishing Co.

MONEY, J. (Ed.) (1962) *Reading Disability: Progress and Research Needs in Dyslexia*. Baltimore: John Hopkins.

MONEY, J. (Ed.) (1966) *The Disabled Reader: Education of the Dyslexic Child*. Baltimore: John Hopkins.

MOYLE, D. (1968) *The Teaching of Reading*. London: Ward Lock Educational.

NAIDOO, S. (1972) *Specific Dyslexia*. I.C.A.A.

NEWTON, M. (1973) *Dyslexia: A Guide for Teachers and Parents*. Birmingham: University of Aston.

TANSLEY, A. E. (1967) *Reading and Remedial Reading*. London: Routledge and Kegan Paul.